Your Personal Fertility Food Tracker Diary

Other Books by the Author:

Dancing Your Way to Fertility
The Infertility Diaries
Your Daily Fertility Success Journal
Super Sperm Your Guy and Beat Infertility So He Can Get You Pregnant:
The Ultimate Male Fertility Preparation Program
Yes, I Can Get Pregnant: Letters for Infertility Patients to Send
Themselves
Perfecting Your Fertility

Visit www.dancingyourwaytofertility.com to learn more!

Your Personal Fertility Food Tracker Diary
Paula Fuoco Davis
PaulaMediaandEntertainment.com, Nashua, NH

ISBN:9781543131024

Edition Notice
Date of Publication: December 21, 2016
Number of Printings: First printing
Year of publication: 2016

Books may be purchased in quantity and/or special sales by contacting the publisher, PaulaMediaandEntertainment.com, dancingyourwaytofertility.com or by email at Frably@aol.com.

Library of Congress Catalog Number:
ISBN:
   1. Infertility 2. Fertility 3. Health

   First Edition

This book is dedicated to my mother, Sarah Fuoco for being the best mother in the world.

My father, Joseph Fuoco, for being one of the kindest men I ever met.

My beautiful children, Amber and Sammy, who God sent as an answer to all my prayers.

Jehovah God, who gives the privilege of prayer and who is always there.

My husband, Christopher Davis, for being there and walking this hard road with me. You were brave and kind, a true hero, and without you, I would not have my kids.

Your Personal Fertility Food Tracker Diary

When working towards healing from infertility, never for one moment underestimate the power of the foods you eat.

Right now, this moment, you need to begin seeing everything you eat and drink as either a potential healer of your infertility or a potential destroyer of your fertility.

The foods you eat right now could mean the difference between getting pregnant and not getting pregnant. This is how important the food component of your fertility journey is.

Do not be fooled into thinking that you can drink lots of coffee, eat white flour products, sugar, and processed, fast-foods and it won't impact your body's ability to conceive.

Yes, there are some women who can live off fast food and still get pregnant whenever they choose—but there are also millions of women whose fertility is being stolen by the foods they eat.

To prepare for pregnancy, it is key that you plan, choose and decide to eat as healthy as possible to maximize your body's ability to have a baby.

Don't be trapped into thinking that you can eat the way you've always eaten and still heal your body.

If getting pregnant is not coming easily to you, you need to change your eating habits and let go of archaic ideas about food that could be holding your body back.

Every time you are tempted by that chocolate bar in the vending machine at work, or a cup of coffee, or a cracker with lots of hydrogenated oil, remind yourself that chocolate bar, or that cup of coffee, or that cracker, could be what ultimately prevents you from having a baby.

If you think a bagel, cream cheese and coffee is a healthy way to start to the day, think again.

It is simple: what you eat can make you weak or make you strong. The right foods can heal your infertility and the wrong ones can rob you of your right to be a mother.

It is important that every day, you keep track of what you eat. How healthy you become is closely related to the foods you take into your body.

There is a direct correlation between your level of fertility, vitality and energy and the foods and liquids you consume.

Ask yourself:

What foods make me feel stronger, brighten my mood, and give me energy?

What foods give me a second wind?

What foods leave me feeling exhausted?

What foods make me tired and cranky?

What live foods do I eat daily?

Breakfast: Say goodbye to cereal and milk, a bagel and coffee, pancakes and maple syrup. Say hello to oatmeal, blueberries and spinach.

Starting your diet with a few teaspoons of cooked spinach, maybe with a pinch or two of romano grated cheese.

Other great breakfast choices: lots of walnuts, avocados and blueberries, a big bowl or romaine lettuce doused with olive oil. A big glass of juiced spinach and kale. A smoothie with spinach, maca, flax seed, blueberries and honey. Or a bowl of walnuts and brazil nuts.

You have to replace all the ideas you've had about traditional breakfast foods, and replace them with foods that are alive, not laden down with corn syrup, sugar and white flour. The standard breakfast foods most of us eat can wreak havoc with our fertility.

The goal each morning should be to eat nuts, beans, vegetables. No more lattes, coffees, or anything else caffeinated, white-floured or sugared to kick-start your day.

Lunch: Say goodbye to fast food lunches, deli meat, or lots of poor quality red meat.

Say hello to salads with things like walnuts and chick peas in them. Say goodbye to caffeine and soda to get through the day. No more chips with that tuna fish sandwich. A healthy lunch could include a salad with some chicken in it, homemade vegetable soup, with an apple, a grilled cheese with whole grain bread. A healthy lunch could also include a pumpkin-sunflower seed combination, or slices of pineapple drizzled with honey. A pita pocket filled with parsley, basil and kale, drizzled with olive oil and flaxseed oil.

Snacks: Snacks should include lots of healthy fruits, seeds, nuts, and vegetables. Candy bars, diet drinks or desserts, sugary desserts, chips, all should be eliminated.

Dinner: No white flour, trans fats, fast food, foods that contain msg or trans fats. Think lean proteins, healthy fish, lots of greens, salad, vegetables, nuts, and olive oil.

Here are some tips that will help you use food as a way to heal your infertility and prepare your body for pregnancy:

To start:

• Stop Or Reduce Your Coffee Consumption

Do you drink coffee? You need to consider stopping. As much as you can, preferably stop all coffee.

If you can't stop, drink no more than a half a cup to a cup a day. That's it. Ideally, do everything you can to say goodbye to coffee for now. Coffee is an enemy of your fertility. Every time you are tempted to drink coffee, remind yourself that this cup of coffee could rob you of the ability to give birth to children. Get rid of all caffeine products in your life. Extreme, maybe, but coffee can weaken key organs, such as the liver, and right now, you need to stack the odds in your favor.

Some studies have shown that women who drink high amounts of coffee take up to three times longer to conceive, and even small amounts of coffee can hamper fertility.

To cope with the lack of coffee in your life, you may need to go to bed earlier and eat healthier to compensate for the energy the coffee gave you to get through the day. Coffee cannot be your fuel or main source of energy anymore. Your energy has to come from healthy foods, vitamins, juices, exercise and other genuinely healthy energy-producing sources.

As you detoxify and strengthen your body, your energy will increase and come from your inner core of health—not coffee, an imposter who pretends to hand you energy, but ultimately steals it. Say goodbye to coffee and hello to food sources that genuinely fuel you.

• Eliminate Most Sugars

Do you eat lots of sweets? Realize that donuts, candy, cake, and other foods with sugar weaken your body and can prevent you from becoming pregnant.

Sugar puts your body in a diseased, acidic state. Sugar can cause hormone imbalances, vitamin deficiencies, high insulin levels, and a compromised immune system. While an occasional sweet is okay, overall you'll want to drastically reduce the sugar in your life.
It can be hard to quit eating all sweets entirely. Many of us have sugar cravings, but overall you want to drastically reduce the amount of sugar you consume.

You'll also need to be be aware and carefully examine the foods you eat that may have hidden sugars in them. Read labels carefully as sugar content varies by brand. Always remember: if its packaged, there is a chance it might have sugar in it.

Foods you need to be aware of for potential sugar content include:

• Yogurt
• Cereals
• Canned vegetables
• Canned soups
• Breakfast bars
• Salad dressing
• Condiments
• White flour products.
• Breads and rolls
• Juices
• Fast foods
• Barbecue sauce
• Soda
• Spaghetti sauce
• Energy drinks
• Dried fruit
• Crackers

• Products that list ingredients such as, dextrose, fructose, corn syrup, high-fructose corn syrup, fruit juice concentrate, lactose, sorbitol, xylitol, maltodetrin and turbinado sugar, polydextrose, mannitol, and turbinado sugar. Ingredients ending in 'ose' is often a likely form of sugar.
• Oatmeal
• Protein bars
• Ice tea
• Ketchup
• Frozen meal entrees, even diet ones
• Syrups
• Jelly and jams
• Fruit juice concentrate
• Bouillon cubes

- Bacon
- Luncheon meats

• Consider Reducing Hydrogenated Oils, Also Known As Trans Fats

Another category of food you need to consider cutting from your diet entirely are foods made with hydrogenated oils, also known as trans fats. Several studies have shown that women with fertility problems eat more trans fats or hydrogenated oils than fertile women. Hydrogenated oil is a man-made food substance used widely throughout the food industry because it lengthens the shelf life of many foods and is cost effective.

Trans fats interfere with the metabolic processes in the body, because they take the place of essential fatty acids that perform critical functions. Trans fats clog up the space that natural fats should occupy, making it difficult for essential nutrients to pass in and out of the cells. Bodily functions are altered by these artificial molecules that enter the system.

Various studies have shown that women who eat a diet high in hydrogenated oils are at increased risk for developing endometriosis.

The World Health Organization has tried to outlaw trans fats for decades.

Some say trans fats work against the body, because they cause a cell-by-cell failure that destroys the flexibility of healthy cell membranes—basically tearing the body down from the inside out.

Trans fats increase bad cholesterol, block production of chemicals that combat inflammation and benefit the body's hormonal and nervous systems. Trans fats are also linked to heart disease, stroke and diabetes.

They interfere with the absorption of essential fatty acids and DHA, and weaken cell walls and compromise cellular structure.

That means, if you are trying to get pregnant, you need to dramatically reduce eating foods made with hydrogenated oils, corn oil, vegetable oil, transfats and corn syrup.

Be sure to read food labels carefully so you are aware of what products contain hydrogenated oils.

Fast food restaurants often serve a lot of foods loaded with hydrogenated oils. Cake, pancake, biscuit, and cookie mixes are usually made with hydrogenated oils.

Diet foods that promise 'no fat' often have hydrogenated oils.

Labels that say partially hydrogenated, or hydrogenated, contain trans fats. Even foods that promise to be trans fat free may contain up to 0.5 grams of partially hydrogenated oil, a source of trans fats.

Remember that if you see the word 'hydrogenated' or partially hydrogenated, it means it contains a trans fat. Hydrogenated oils are also trans fats, and that includes hydrogenated coconut or soybean oil.

Read labels carefully because hydrogenated oil content can vary by brand.

Begin to replace hydrogenated oils with healthy oils your body needs, such as olive oil, coconut oil and flax seed oil.

It is best to avoid as many pre-packaged foods that you can at this time. Foods to be aware of can include:

• Commercially baked cakes, cookies, muffins, pies, donuts
• Crackers
• Peanut butter
• Frozen meals
• Frozen bakery items
• French fries
• Whipped toppings
• Margarines

- Shortening
- Cake frosting
- Taco shells
- Microwave popcorn
- Breakfast cereals
- Corn chips and potato chips
- Frozen pizzas and frozen burritos
- Low-fat ice creams
- Pre-made noodle soups and soup mixes
- Bread
- Pasta mixes
- Sauce mixes
- Deep fried foods
- Frozen breakfast foods
- Packaged snacks
- Many different types of candies
- Some salted peanuts
- White bread
- Non-dairy creamers
- Tortillas
- Donuts
- Peanut butter
- Ice cream and low fat ice cream
- Hamburger and hot dog buns
- Movie popcorn
- Frozen pizza
- Refrigerated dough products
- Most fried foods—ask what type of oil the product is fried in
- Piecrust
- Cake mixes
- Pancakes and pancake mixes
- Waffles
- Frozen burgers
- Beef hot dogs
- Refrigerated cookie dough
- Biscuits and sweet rolls
- Refrigerated dough
- Breakfast sandwiches
- Meat sticks

- Crunchy noodles
- Canned chili
- Packaged pudding
- Fish sticks
- Low-fat ice cream
- Frozen burritos
- Noodle soup cups
- Cocoa or hot chocolate mix
- Instant mashed potatoes
- Gravy mixes
- Dips
- Potato chips
- Frozen pot pies
- Sandwiches grilled at a restaurant
- Reduced fat and fat free noodles
- Spreads

• Consider Eliminating Alcohol

At this time, it is best to stop all alcohol. A glass of wine occasionally when trying to get pregnant might not hurt, but nothing more and no hard liquors. Many studies suggest that the higher your alcohol consumption, the less chance you have of conceiving. Alcohol can impair the detoxifying process that occurs within the liver, and if the liver is working hard to metabolize alcohol, it can become run down and sick. Too much alcohol can also contribute to hormonal imbalances.

Alcohol can adversely affect ovulation and affect the body's ability to produce the amino acids necessary for cell development.

• Cut Down On White Flour Products

How many white flour products do you eat each day? Do you start your day with a bagel, donut or white bread toast? If so, get rid of white flour in your life as much as possible. An occasional bowl of spaghetti may be okay, but in general, you want to reduce the white flour products in your life as much as you can. White flour products, including pasta, bagels and bread, are not health builders and will not advance your goal of becoming pregnant.

If you feel extremely weak and lethargic after eating white flour products, you may have celiac disease or a wheat intolerance. Symptoms include stomachaches, fatigue, bloating and flatulence. Check labels and brands. Some sources of white flour can include:

- Alcohol
- Crackers
- Cereals
- Corn flour
- Cake and cookie mixes
- Pancake mixes
- Muffin mixes
- Puddings
- Pretzels
- Donuts
- Foods with artificial colorings and preservatives
- Sweet and sour glazes
- Sweet sauces
- Soy sauce
- Ice cream cones
- Foods containing malt
- Powdered or canned soups
- Fast foods
- Gravies

Instead, choose wheat-free products made from rice, oat, rye, and puffed rice cereals.

• Reduce Your Intake Of Diet Foods or Foods with Sugar Substitutes

You may want to consider reducing your intake of diet foods, diet drinks or foods with sugar substitutes or artificial sweeteners. Some experts on fertility recommend avoiding sweeteners listed on labels as aspartame, sucralose, acesulfame potassium, also listed as acesulfame k and ACE, neotame, and saccharin.

Consider cutting back or eliminating diet drinks and powdered drinks that contain any of these sweeteners.

These sweeteners may also be in some chewing gums and ice creams.

Some doctors have concluded that these artificial sweeteners interfere with fetal development, and act as 'instant birth control.' Aspartame is considered a endocrine disrupting chemical, by some medical providers.

Artificial sweeteners and sugar substitutes negatively impact the hormones in the pituitary glands, thyroid and ovaries.

Hidden sources of these artificial sweeteners can include:

- Breads
- Jello
- Gelatins
- Toothpaste
- Breath mints
- Drink mixes
- Syrups
- Jellies
- Cereals
- Sugar-free candies

• Reduce or Eliminate Soy

Some studies suggest that high levels of soy act as endocrine disrupters and decrease fertility. The phytoestrogens found in soy interfere with endocrine function and can mimic the female hormone oestrogen, which disrupts the normal production of sex hormones. Soy can decrease the follicle-stimulating hormone (FSH), as well as the leutinizing hormone.

Many soy products are genetically engineered and can reduce the body's ability to absorb minerals. Some soy isoflavones mimic estrogen— which means the body thinks it has estrogen it doesn't have, thus causing hormone imbalances. Some studies have also shown that soy can lead to thyroid problems, such as hypothyroidism.

Soy derivatives are often labeled under different names, including mono-diglyceride, soya, soja, yuba, TSF or textured soy flour, TSP textured soy protein, TVP textured vegetable protein, lecithin, and MSG, yeast extract, soy protein.

Hidden sources of soy include:

- Protein bars
- Meal replacement shakes
- Bottled fruit drinks
- Soups
- Sauces
- Baked goods
- Breakfast cereals
- Chewing gum
- Chocolate
- Bread
- Microwave meals
- Frozen pizzas
- Processed meat
- Soy milk
- Soy beans
- Corn chips
- Canned tuna

• Avoid Fish Known To Potentially Have High Mercury Levels

Due to high mercury levels, some types of fish are best avoided or eaten rarely when trying to get pregnant. These include swordfish, shark, grouper, marlin, orange roughy, tilefish, mackerel, tuna, bluefish, lobster, halibut, croaker and bass saltwater.

The fish with the reported lowest amounts of mercury include calamari, crab, pollock, scallops, salmon, shrimp, clams, and others, but these also need to be eaten in moderation.

• No MSG

Avoid foods that could have monosodium glutamate, also known as MSG. Foods that might contain MSG include potato chips, Chinese food, meat seasonings and packaged soups. MSG can appear on labels as autolyzed yeast, maltodextrin, hydrolyzed pea protein.

• Other Foods To Avoid

• Avoid raw or undercooked meats.
• Avoid raw or undercooked eggs.
• Stay Away From Fast Food
• Avoid Deli Meats

Fertility-Strengthening Foods

• Eat More Vegetables

Here's a simple fact that will increase your fertility: the more vegetables you eat, the more fertile you will be.

Repeat: More vegetables you eat, the healthier and more fertile you will be. Implant that thought in your brain, please, please, please.

Your diet should include a lot of vegetables every single day.

Note the word: a lot.

In fact, most of the foods you eat, starting with breakfast, should be vegetables.

Starting now, the way you eat should revolve around vegetables.

Vegetables should no longer be just a small side dish you include with dinner—they should be the main course, present at almost every meal and every snack you eat. They are the key to healing your body. You need to start looking at vegetables in a way that is not traditional in our culture—as your main source of food.

Vegetables should become part of your breakfast, your snacks, lunch and dinner. You want to find as many ways as you can to dramatically increase the vegetables you eat daily.

For lunch, eat a big bowl of romaine lettuce. Munch on parsley for a snack. Roast some asparagus and olive oil to eat before bed. Bake some sweet potatoes and olive oil for snack. Include spinach in your salads or sandwiches.

Slice up some peppers, carrots, red and green peppers, tomatoes, and seaweeds and place in bags so you have easy-to-eat snacks ready throughout the day.

Don't allow a busy schedule to force you to have to run to the nearest fast food drive-through because you are starving and need to just fill your stomach. At night before bed, prepare a salad of chicory and romaine lettuce. Or just wash some kale or spinach, put in a bag, and have it on your way home from work.

Nibble on broccoli before bed. Include a salad with every meal. Put vegetables on your pizza, in your tomato sauces, soups and stews.

Instead of a sandwich of deli meat, how about a sandwich of tomato and basil, broccoli and cheese, or spinach and tomato?

Eat vegetables the way you would eat fruit—a whole cucumber, a whole tomato, a whole carrot.

Select one or two days a week and eat only vegetables the entire day. Start your day with a green veggie drink or smoothie, add some flaxseed, coconut oil, maca, honey and spirulina.

Make a vegetable breakfast wrap, top an multi-grain English muffin with onions, peppers, and tomatoes. Create dips with vegetables—and then dip your vegetables! Add vegetables to spreads like hummus or mashed avocados. Make vegetable submarine sandwiches, with healthy bread and lots of olive oil.

Juicing or smoothies are a great way to include more vegetables in your diet. Drink a glass of spinach juice each day. Juice parsley, kale, beets, and garlic once or twice a day.

Start including garlic in many of your recipes as you can. Chew on garlic, juice garlic and make garlic part of your daily eating routine.

Remember: from now on, vegetables should make up more than 60 to 70 percent of the foods you eat each day.

Some super fertility vegetables include:

• Spinach is high in iron and folic acid, two important nutrients for reproductive health. Women with low iron intakes are at greater risk for ovulatory fertility.

To enhance absorption of iron from spinach, combine it with a food that contains vitamin C, such as broccoli, strawberries, green peppers or oranges.

• Alfalfa provides the body with a rich source of essential minerals important for reproductive health.

• Broccoli and cabbage contain a phytonutrient that helps with estrogen metabolism.

• Yams and sweet potatoes contain a compound called diosgenins which impacts hormonal patterns and increases ovulation. Yams have massive amounts of vitamin A that improve cervical fluid and follicle development. They are also loaded with beta carotene that helps regulate the menstrual cycle. It also has high amounts of Vitamin B which helps regulate hormones. They also help stabilize blood sugar— and the more stable your sugar levels, the better your ovulation will be.

• Asparagus is also a high fertility food.

• Wheat Grass is one of the best sources of living chlorophyll. It helps balance the PH levels in the body and is high in magnesium, which helps restore sex hormones.

• Spirulina is a great source of the essential acid GLA.

• Chlorella: a green algae that helps the body cleanse and detoxify.

Here is a checklist to help you keep track of the vegetables you eat each day:

Vegetables to eat every day include:

--Spinach
--Yams and Sweet Potatoes
--Peppers
--Broccoli
--Arugula
--Asparagus
--Romaine
--Seaweed
--Garlic
--Cabbage
--Dandelion greens
--Romaine Lettuce
--Red Peppers
--Dark green lettuce
--Kale
--Asparagus
--Beets
--Seaweeds
--Brussel sprouts

• Eat More Fruits

Along with eating as many vegetables as possible, start including more fruits in your diet.

Fruits are packed with antioxidants, which protect the body from cell aging and damage—including cells in the reproductive system, like your eggs.

Start eating one or two bowls of blueberries for breakfast. Blueberries have phytonutrients that have hormone balancing properties that impact ovulation.

Many holistic practitioners recommend eating avocados to boost fertility, because they are a great source of Vitamin E, a huge fertility booster. Avocados help regulate both ovulation and production of cervical mucus. They are rich in folic acid and vitamin B6, which helps prevent luteal phase defect.

Bananas are full of potassium, Vitamin C and fiber, and bromelain which increases sex hormone production.

Slice up some papaya as your bedtime snack, have two or three bowls of strawberries, blackberries, raspberries and blueberries for breakfast, bring apples to work.

Eat fresh pineapple daily, including the pineapple core. Pineapple contains bromelain that aids in implantation. Pineapple is also one the best natural sources of manganese, an important mineral that triggers production of various reproductive hormones. Low levels of this mineral have been reported to be associated with difficulty conceiving. Note: if you are already taking aspirin, be aware that pineapple might thin your blood.

Pomegranates are considered a fertility super food.

Eat lots of fruits that contain Vitamin C, such as oranges, kiwi, blueberries and strawberries, a nutrient key to fertile health.

Fruits to include in your daily diet:

-Plums
-Blueberries
-Strawberries
-Bananas
-Grapes
-Cantaloupe
-Oranges
-Apples
-Mangoes
-Bananas
-Blueberries
-Lemons
-Pomegranate
-Figs
-Apricots
-Prunes
-Peaches
-Blackberries

• Eat More Beans

Beans are an essential food for developing good follicle quality. Black beans are considered by some to be a reproductive tonic. Lentils are also a healthy source of iron that support ovulation and aid fertility. Aduki beans are considered to support the Kidney Qi, which is essential for reproductive function.

• Eat More Nuts

Start including lots of nuts in your diet, such as walnuts, almonds, and brazil nuts. Nuts have high amounts of Omega 3 and Omega 6, which have been known to improve sperm quality and egg quality.

Nuts can enhance pancreas function, thus helping to regulate insulin and blood sugar levels in the body. Almonds contain L-arginine and zinc which are important nutrients to the reproductive system. Walnuts are high in protein and folic acid and are an excellent source of omega-3 fatty acids. Almonds contain high levels of zinc and L-arginine, which are important nutrients to the reproductive system.

• Eat More Seeds

Seeds contain a lot of omega 3s which are key to fertility. Pumpkin seeds which contain zinc, an important nutrient in egg production. Sunflower seeds and sesame seeds provide healthy fats. Black sesame seeds can help enhance liver function and sesame seeds are rich in minerals.

• Healthy Oils

Because fat intake is so vital to fertility, include olive oil, coconut oil and flaxseed oil in your diet. Healthy fats, as opposed to trans fats, can make the body more fertile, reduce inflammation in the body and increase insulin sensitivity.

Olive oil, like avocados, has monounsaturated fat, which helps assist in reproduction. Some people have taken a mixture of olive oil, honey and mustard seed to enhance their fertility.

Flax seed oil helps the hormones hit the receptor cells in a precise way so they can work at their maximum capacity. This helps the membranes in the receptor cells be more flexible, run more smoothly and makes it easier for hormones to bind with. It also encourages healing in the uterus, and is rich in omega fatty acids.

Coconut oil helps maintain hormonal balance for reproduction and helps thyroid function and ovulation cycles.

• Honey

Bee pollen stimulates ovarian function. It is also rich in minerals such as copper, potassium, and zinc and also has 20 of the 22 known amino acids. Bee pollen contains natural hormonal substances that stimulate and nourish the reproductive system, stimulate ovarian function and increase the health and biological value of the egg.

• Wild Salmon

According to Chinese medicine, salmon is good for nourishing the yin and blood, helping to generate healthy follicles and ample amounts of cervical fluid.

• Lean Cuts of Meat

When possible, choose lean cuts of meat. An overload of heavy red meat can work against your fertility.

• Drink Lots of Good Quality Water

Drinking a lot of the right water can do so much to enhance your fertility. Water increases cervical fluid which is key in conception. Water can help sperm stay alive for days. Water also facilitates the transport of hormones and plumps up follicles.

The key is that along with drinking a lot of water, you need to drink high-quality water. Do you drink tap water? What is the quality of the water in your community? For now, start buying purified water and use it for all your drinking and cooking needs. Put a filter on your tap water. As much as you can, stop drinking water out of plastic bottles that can contain the chemical bisphenol A, also known as BPA. Keep your water stored in glass containers, rather than plastic.

• Start Your Day Drinking Lemon in Warm Water

Lemon enhances your immunity and increases liver and digestive health.

• Brown Rice

Replace white rice with brown rice for enhanced nutrition. Brown rice is a slow carbohydrate, which means a gradual rise in blood sugar after being eaten.

• Green Tea

For better quality eggs and more viable embryos, consider drinking two or more cups of green tea a day. Green tea contains polyphenols and hypoxanthine, which increase the percentage of viable embryos. Hypoxanthine enhances the follicular fluid that helps eggs mature and be ready for fertilization.

Green tea also contains polyhenols that act as an antioxidant and gets rid of unwanted toxins in the body. Green tea can help repair oxidative damage that occurs in the body due to stress, aging and the environment. Drink in moderation, as it can decrease the body's absorption of iron and decrease the effects of folic acid, so you might want to make sure you taking adequate amounts of iron and folic acid at the same time.

You should reduce the amount of green tea you drink once you are pregnant or if there is even a slight chance you are pregnant. The polyphenols in green tea that help prevent chromosomal abnormalities in your eggs can cause an embryo to miscarry or fail to implant.

• Pomegranates and Natural Pomegranate Juice

Pomegranates help boost fertility by increasing blood flow to the uterus and thickening the uterine lining. They also help balance the hormones estrogen and progesterone.

The antioxidants in pomegranates help prevent DNA damage to eggs and contain folic acid, essential during the early stages of a pregnancy.

• Pineapple Core

Cut the core into round sections and eat after embryo transfers to help implantation. The bromelain found in the core reduces inflammation and improves uterine lining.

• Brewer's Yeast

Brewer's yeast is a great source of B complex, and is rich in minerals like zinc, iron and chromium.

Your Personal Fertility Food Tracker Diary

Today's Date:

Green Foods Eaten Today:

Fruits Eaten Today:

Vegetables Eaten Today:

Nuts Eaten Today:

Seeds Eaten Today:

Healthy Oils Eaten Today:

Vegetable and/or Fruit Drinks Made Today:

Vitamin and Herb Supplements:

Glasses of high-quality, filtered or bottled water:

Check if You Ate:
Spinach
Strawberries
Broccoli
Bee Pollen
Alfalfa
Green Tea
Artichokes
Cabbage
Yams
Sweet Potatoes
Asparagus
Spirulina
Chlorella
Wheat Grass
Romaine lettuce
Seaweed
Garlic
Dandelion greens
Red peppers
Kale
Beets
Blueberries
Avocados
Apples
Pineapple
Bananas
Pomegranates
Plums
Grapes
Lemons
Brazil Nuts
Walnuts
Almonds
Pumpkin Seeds
Sunflower Seeds
Sesame Seeds
Black Sesame Seeds
Olive Oil

Check if you ate:
Flaxseed Oil
Coconut Oil
Honey
Green Tea

Avoided: (Check off when you said no to)
Coffee
Sugar
Transfats
White Flour products
Alcohol
Soda
Processed Foods
Canned Foods
Diet Foods
Foods that contain transfats
Vegetable Oil and other hydrogenated oils
Soy
Products put on your body that contain chemicals
Sugar substitutes

Today's Date:

Green Foods Eaten Today:

Fruits Eaten Today:

Vegetables Eaten Today:

Nuts Eaten Today:

Seeds Eaten Today:

Healthy Oils Eaten Today:

Vegetable and/or Fruit Drinks Made Today:

Vitamin and Herb Supplements:

Glasses of high-quality, filtered or bottled water:

Check if You Ate:
Spinach
Strawberries
Broccoli
Bee Pollen
Alfalfa
Green Tea
Artichokes
Cabbage
Yams
Sweet Potatoes
Asparagus
Spirulina
Chlorella
Wheat Grass
Romaine lettuce
Seaweed
Garlic
Dandelion greens
Red peppers
Kale
Beets
Blueberries
Avocados
Apples
Pineapple
Bananas
Pomegranates
Plums
Grapes
Lemons
Brazil Nuts
Walnuts
Almonds
Pumpkin Seeds
Sunflower Seeds
Sesame Seeds
Black Sesame Seeds
Olive Oil

Check if you ate:
Flaxseed Oil
Coconut Oil
Honey
Green Tea

Avoided: (Check off when you said no to)
Coffee
Sugar
Transfats
White Flour products
Alcohol
Soda
Processed Foods
Canned Foods
Diet Foods
Foods that contain transfats
Vegetable Oil and other hydrogenated oils
Soy
Products put on your body that contain chemicals
Sugar substitutes

Today's Date:

Green Foods Eaten Today:

Fruits Eaten Today:

Vegetables Eaten Today:

Nuts Eaten Today:

Seeds Eaten Today:

Healthy Oils Eaten Today:

Vegetable and/or Fruit Drinks Made Today:

Vitamin and Herb Supplements:

Glasses of high-quality, filtered or bottled water:

Check if You Ate:

Spinach
Strawberries
Broccoli
Bee Pollen
Alfalfa
Green Tea
Artichokes
Cabbage
Yams
Sweet Potatoes
Asparagus
Spirulina
Chlorella
Wheat Grass
Romaine lettuce
Seaweed
Garlic
Dandelion greens
Red peppers
Kale
Beets
Blueberries
Avocados
Apples
Pineapple
Bananas
Pomegranates
Plums
Grapes
Lemons
Brazil Nuts
Walnuts
Almonds
Pumpkin Seeds
Sunflower Seeds
Sesame Seeds
Black Sesame Seeds
Olive Oil

Check if you ate:
Flaxseed Oil
Coconut Oil
Honey
Green Tea

Avoided: (Check off when you said no to)
Coffee
Sugar
Transfats
White Flour products
Alcohol
Soda
Processed Foods
Canned Foods
Diet Foods
Foods that contain transfats
Vegetable Oil and other hydrogenated oils
Soy
Products put on your body that contain chemicals
Sugar substitutes

Today's Date:

Green Foods Eaten Today:

Fruits Eaten Today:

Vegetables Eaten Today:

Nuts Eaten Today:

Seeds Eaten Today:

Healthy Oils Eaten Today:

Vegetable and/or Fruit Drinks Made Today:

Vitamin and Herb Supplements:

Glasses of high-quality, filtered or bottled water:

Check if You Ate:

Spinach
Strawberries
Broccoli
Bee Pollen
Alfalfa
Green Tea
Artichokes
Cabbage
Yams
Sweet Potatoes
Asparagus
Spirulina
Chlorella
Wheat Grass
Romaine lettuce
Seaweed
Garlic
Dandelion greens
Red peppers
Kale
Beets
Blueberries
Avocados
Apples
Pineapple
Bananas
Pomegranates
Plums
Grapes
Lemons
Brazil Nuts
Walnuts
Almonds
Pumpkin Seeds
Sunflower Seeds
Sesame Seeds
Black Sesame Seeds
Olive Oil

Check if you ate:
Flaxseed Oil
Coconut Oil
Honey
Green Tea

Avoided: (Check off when you said no to)
Coffee
Sugar
Transfats
White Flour products
Alcohol
Soda
Processed Foods
Canned Foods
Diet Foods
Foods that contain transfats
Vegetable Oil and other hydrogenated oils
Soy
Products put on your body that contain chemicals
Sugar substitutes

Today's Date:

Green Foods Eaten Today:

Fruits Eaten Today:

Vegetables Eaten Today:

Nuts Eaten Today:

Seeds Eaten Today:

Healthy Oils Eaten Today:

Vegetable and/or Fruit Drinks Made Today:

Vitamin and Herb Supplements:

Glasses of high-quality, filtered or bottled water:

Check if You Ate:
Spinach
Strawberries
Broccoli
Bee Pollen
Alfalfa
Green Tea
Artichokes
Cabbage
Yams
Sweet Potatoes
Asparagus
Spirulina
Chlorella
Wheat Grass
Romaine lettuce
Seaweed
Garlic
Dandelion greens
Red peppers
Kale
Beets
Blueberries
Avocados
Apples
Pineapple
Bananas
Pomegranates
Plums
Grapes
Lemons
Brazil Nuts
Walnuts
Almonds
Pumpkin Seeds
Sunflower Seeds
Sesame Seeds
Black Sesame Seeds
Olive Oil

Check if you ate:
Flaxseed Oil
Coconut Oil
Honey
Green Tea

Avoided: (Check off when you said no to)
Coffee
Sugar
Transfats
White Flour products
Alcohol
Soda
Processed Foods
Canned Foods
Diet Foods
Foods that contain transfats
Vegetable Oil and other hydrogenated oils
Soy
Products put on your body that contain chemicals
Sugar substitutes

Today's Date:

Green Foods Eaten Today:

Fruits Eaten Today:

Vegetables Eaten Today:

Nuts Eaten Today:

Seeds Eaten Today:

Healthy Oils Eaten Today:

Vegetable and/or Fruit Drinks Made Today:

Vitamin and Herb Supplements:

Glasses of high-quality, filtered or bottled water:

Check if You Ate:
Spinach
Strawberries
Broccoli
Bee Pollen
Alfalfa
Green Tea
Artichokes
Cabbage
Yams
Sweet Potatoes
Asparagus
Spirulina
Chlorella
Wheat Grass
Romaine lettuce
Seaweed
Garlic
Dandelion greens
Red peppers
Kale
Beets
Blueberries
Avocados
Apples
Pineapple
Bananas
Pomegranates
Plums
Grapes
Lemons
Brazil Nuts
Walnuts
Almonds
Pumpkin Seeds
Sunflower Seeds
Sesame Seeds
Black Sesame Seeds
Olive Oil

Check if you ate:
Flaxseed Oil
Coconut Oil
Honey
Green Tea

Avoided: (Check off when you said no to)
Coffee
Sugar
Transfats
White Flour products
Alcohol
Soda
Processed Foods
Canned Foods
Diet Foods
Foods that contain transfats
Vegetable Oil and other hydrogenated oils
Soy
Products put on your body that contain chemicals
Sugar substitutes

Today's Date:

Green Foods Eaten Today:

Fruits Eaten Today:

Vegetables Eaten Today:

Nuts Eaten Today:

Seeds Eaten Today:

Healthy Oils Eaten Today:

Vegetable and/or Fruit Drinks Made Today:

Vitamin and Herb Supplements:

Glasses of high-quality, filtered or bottled water:

Check if You Ate:
Spinach
Strawberries
Broccoli
Bee Pollen
Alfalfa
Green Tea
Artichokes
Cabbage
Yams
Sweet Potatoes
Asparagus
Spirulina
Chlorella
Wheat Grass
Romaine lettuce
Seaweed
Garlic
Dandelion greens
Red peppers
Kale
Beets
Blueberries
Avocados
Apples
Pineapple
Bananas
Pomegranates
Plums
Grapes
Lemons
Brazil Nuts
Walnuts
Almonds
Pumpkin Seeds
Sunflower Seeds
Sesame Seeds
Black Sesame Seeds
Olive Oil

Check if you ate:
Flaxseed Oil
Coconut Oil
Honey
Green Tea

Avoided: (Check off when you said no to)
Coffee
Sugar
Transfats
White Flour products
Alcohol
Soda
Processed Foods
Canned Foods
Diet Foods
Foods that contain transfats
Vegetable Oil and other hydrogenated oils
Soy
Products put on your body that contain chemicals
Sugar substitutes

Today's Date:

Green Foods Eaten Today:

Fruits Eaten Today:

Vegetables Eaten Today:

Nuts Eaten Today:

Seeds Eaten Today:

Healthy Oils Eaten Today:

Vegetable and/or Fruit Drinks Made Today:

Vitamin and Herb Supplements:

Glasses of high-quality, filtered or bottled water:

Check if You Ate:
Spinach
Strawberries
Broccoli
Bee Pollen
Alfalfa
Green Tea
Artichokes
Cabbage
Yams
Sweet Potatoes
Asparagus
Spirulina
Chlorella
Wheat Grass
Romaine lettuce
Seaweed
Garlic
Dandelion greens
Red peppers
Kale
Beets
Blueberries
Avocados
Apples
Pineapple
Bananas
Pomegranates
Plums
Grapes
Lemons
Brazil Nuts
Walnuts
Almonds
Pumpkin Seeds
Sunflower Seeds
Sesame Seeds
Black Sesame Seeds
Olive Oil

Check if you ate:
Flaxseed Oil
Coconut Oil
Honey
Green Tea

Avoided: (Check off when you said no to)
Coffee
Sugar
Transfats
White Flour products
Alcohol
Soda
Processed Foods
Canned Foods
Diet Foods
Foods that contain transfats
Vegetable Oil and other hydrogenated oils
Soy
Products put on your body that contain chemicals
Sugar substitutes

Today's Date:

Green Foods Eaten Today:

Fruits Eaten Today:

Vegetables Eaten Today:

Nuts Eaten Today:

Seeds Eaten Today:

Healthy Oils Eaten Today:

Vegetable and/or Fruit Drinks Made Today:

Vitamin and Herb Supplements:

Glasses of high-quality, filtered or bottled water:

Check if You Ate:
Spinach
Strawberries
Broccoli
Bee Pollen
Alfalfa
Green Tea
Artichokes
Cabbage
Yams
Sweet Potatoes
Asparagus
Spirulina
Chlorella
Wheat Grass
Romaine lettuce
Seaweed
Garlic
Dandelion greens
Red peppers
Kale
Beets
Blueberries
Avocados
Apples
Pineapple
Bananas
Pomegranates
Plums
Grapes
Lemons
Brazil Nuts
Walnuts
Almonds
Pumpkin Seeds
Sunflower Seeds
Sesame Seeds
Black Sesame Seeds
Olive Oil

Check if you ate:
Flaxseed Oil
Coconut Oil
Honey
Green Tea

Avoided: (Check off when you said no to)
Coffee
Sugar
Transfats
White Flour products
Alcohol
Soda
Processed Foods
Canned Foods
Diet Foods
Foods that contain transfats
Vegetable Oil and other hydrogenated oils
Soy
Products put on your body that contain chemicals
Sugar substitutes

Today's Date:

Green Foods Eaten Today:

Fruits Eaten Today:

Vegetables Eaten Today:

Nuts Eaten Today:

Seeds Eaten Today:

Healthy Oils Eaten Today:

Vegetable and/or Fruit Drinks Made Today:

Vitamin and Herb Supplements:

Glasses of high-quality, filtered or bottled water:

Check if You Ate:
Spinach
Strawberries
Broccoli
Bee Pollen
Alfalfa
Green Tea
Artichokes
Cabbage
Yams
Sweet Potatoes
Asparagus
Spirulina
Chlorella
Wheat Grass
Romaine lettuce
Seaweed
Garlic
Dandelion greens
Red peppers
Kale
Beets
Blueberries
Avocados
Apples
Pineapple
Bananas
Pomegranates
Plums
Grapes
Lemons
Brazil Nuts
Walnuts
Almonds
Pumpkin Seeds
Sunflower Seeds
Sesame Seeds
Black Sesame Seeds
Olive Oil

Check if you ate:
Flaxseed Oil
Coconut Oil
Honey
Green Tea

Avoided: (Check off when you said no to)
Coffee
Sugar
Transfats
White Flour products
Alcohol
Soda
Processed Foods
Canned Foods
Diet Foods
Foods that contain transfats
Vegetable Oil and other hydrogenated oils
Soy
Products put on your body that contain chemicals
Sugar substitutes

Today's Date:

Green Foods Eaten Today:

Fruits Eaten Today:

Vegetables Eaten Today:

Nuts Eaten Today:

Seeds Eaten Today:

Healthy Oils Eaten Today:

Vegetable and/or Fruit Drinks Made Today:

Vitamin and Herb Supplements:

Glasses of high-quality, filtered or bottled water:

Check if You Ate:
Spinach
Strawberries
Broccoli
Bee Pollen
Alfalfa
Green Tea
Artichokes
Cabbage
Yams
Sweet Potatoes
Asparagus
Spirulina
Chlorella
Wheat Grass
Romaine lettuce
Seaweed
Garlic
Dandelion greens
Red peppers
Kale
Beets
Blueberries
Avocados
Apples
Pineapple
Bananas
Pomegranates
Plums
Grapes
Lemons
Brazil Nuts
Walnuts
Almonds
Pumpkin Seeds
Sunflower Seeds
Sesame Seeds
Black Sesame Seeds
Olive Oil

Check if you ate:
Flaxseed Oil
Coconut Oil
Honey
Green Tea

Avoided: (Check off when you said no to)
Coffee
Sugar
Transfats
White Flour products
Alcohol
Soda
Processed Foods
Canned Foods
Diet Foods
Foods that contain transfats
Vegetable Oil and other hydrogenated oils
Soy
Products put on your body that contain chemicals
Sugar substitutes

Today's Date:

Green Foods Eaten Today:

Fruits Eaten Today:

Vegetables Eaten Today:

Nuts Eaten Today:

Seeds Eaten Today:

Healthy Oils Eaten Today:

Vegetable and/or Fruit Drinks Made Today:

Vitamin and Herb Supplements:

Glasses of high-quality, filtered or bottled water:

Check if You Ate:
Spinach
Strawberries
Broccoli
Bee Pollen
Alfalfa
Green Tea
Artichokes
Cabbage
Yams
Sweet Potatoes
Asparagus
Spirulina
Chlorella
Wheat Grass
Romaine lettuce
Seaweed
Garlic
Dandelion greens
Red peppers
Kale
Beets
Blueberries
Avocados
Apples
Pineapple
Bananas
Pomegranates
Plums
Grapes
Lemons
Brazil Nuts
Walnuts
Almonds
Pumpkin Seeds
Sunflower Seeds
Sesame Seeds
Black Sesame Seeds
Olive Oil

Check if you ate:
Flaxseed Oil
Coconut Oil
Honey
Green Tea

Avoided: (Check off when you said no to)
Coffee
Sugar
Transfats
White Flour products
Alcohol
Soda
Processed Foods
Canned Foods
Diet Foods
Foods that contain transfats
Vegetable Oil and other hydrogenated oils
Soy
Products put on your body that contain chemicals
Sugar substitutes

Today's Date:

Green Foods Eaten Today:

Fruits Eaten Today:

Vegetables Eaten Today:

Nuts Eaten Today:

Seeds Eaten Today:

Healthy Oils Eaten Today:

Vegetable and/or Fruit Drinks Made Today:

Vitamin and Herb Supplements:

Glasses of high-quality, filtered or bottled water:

Check if You Ate:
Spinach
Strawberries
Broccoli
Bee Pollen
Alfalfa
Green Tea
Artichokes
Cabbage
Yams
Sweet Potatoes
Asparagus
Spirulina
Chlorella
Wheat Grass
Romaine lettuce
Seaweed
Garlic
Dandelion greens
Red peppers
Kale
Beets
Blueberries
Avocados
Apples
Pineapple
Bananas
Pomegranates
Plums
Grapes
Lemons
Brazil Nuts
Walnuts
Almonds
Pumpkin Seeds
Sunflower Seeds
Sesame Seeds
Black Sesame Seeds
Olive Oil

Check if you ate:
Flaxseed Oil
Coconut Oil
Honey
Green Tea

Avoided: (Check off when you said no to)
Coffee
Sugar
Transfats
White Flour products
Alcohol
Soda
Processed Foods
Canned Foods
Diet Foods
Foods that contain transfats
Vegetable Oil and other hydrogenated oils
Soy
Products put on your body that contain chemicals
Sugar substitutes

Today's Date:

Green Foods Eaten Today:

Fruits Eaten Today:

Vegetables Eaten Today:

Nuts Eaten Today:

Seeds Eaten Today:

Healthy Oils Eaten Today:

Vegetable and/or Fruit Drinks Made Today:

Vitamin and Herb Supplements:

Glasses of high-quality, filtered or bottled water:

Check if You Ate:
Spinach
Strawberries
Broccoli
Bee Pollen
Alfalfa
Green Tea
Artichokes
Cabbage
Yams
Sweet Potatoes
Asparagus
Spirulina
Chlorella
Wheat Grass
Romaine lettuce
Seaweed
Garlic
Dandelion greens
Red peppers
Kale
Beets
Blueberries
Avocados
Apples
Pineapple
Bananas
Pomegranates
Plums
Grapes
Lemons
Brazil Nuts
Walnuts
Almonds
Pumpkin Seeds
Sunflower Seeds
Sesame Seeds
Black Sesame Seeds
Olive Oil

Check if you ate:
Flaxseed Oil
Coconut Oil
Honey
Green Tea

Avoided: (Check off when you said no to)
Coffee
Sugar
Transfats
White Flour products
Alcohol
Soda
Processed Foods
Canned Foods
Diet Foods
Foods that contain transfats
Vegetable Oil and other hydrogenated oils
Soy
Products put on your body that contain chemicals
Sugar substitutes

Today's Date:

Green Foods Eaten Today:

Fruits Eaten Today:

Vegetables Eaten Today:

Nuts Eaten Today:

Seeds Eaten Today:

Healthy Oils Eaten Today:

Vegetable and/or Fruit Drinks Made Today:

Vitamin and Herb Supplements:

Glasses of high-quality, filtered or bottled water:

Check if You Ate:
Spinach
Strawberries
Broccoli
Bee Pollen
Alfalfa
Green Tea
Artichokes
Cabbage
Yams
Sweet Potatoes
Asparagus
Spirulina
Chlorella
Wheat Grass
Romaine lettuce
Seaweed
Garlic
Dandelion greens
Red peppers
Kale
Beets
Blueberries
Avocados
Apples
Pineapple
Bananas
Pomegranates
Plums
Grapes
Lemons
Brazil Nuts
Walnuts
Almonds
Pumpkin Seeds
Sunflower Seeds
Sesame Seeds
Black Sesame Seeds
Olive Oil

Check if you ate:
Flaxseed Oil
Coconut Oil
Honey
Green Tea

Avoided: (Check off when you said no to)
Coffee
Sugar
Transfats
White Flour products
Alcohol
Soda
Processed Foods
Canned Foods
Diet Foods
Foods that contain transfats
Vegetable Oil and other hydrogenated oils
Soy
Products put on your body that contain chemicals
Sugar substitutes

Today's Date:

Green Foods Eaten Today:

Fruits Eaten Today:

Vegetables Eaten Today:

Nuts Eaten Today:

Seeds Eaten Today:

Healthy Oils Eaten Today:

Vegetable and/or Fruit Drinks Made Today:

Vitamin and Herb Supplements:

Glasses of high-quality, filtered or bottled water:

Check if You Ate:
Spinach
Strawberries
Broccoli
Bee Pollen
Alfalfa
Green Tea
Artichokes
Cabbage
Yams
Sweet Potatoes
Asparagus
Spirulina
Chlorella
Wheat Grass
Romaine lettuce
Seaweed
Garlic
Dandelion greens
Red peppers
Kale
Beets
Blueberries
Avocados
Apples
Pineapple
Bananas
Pomegranates
Plums
Grapes
Lemons
Brazil Nuts
Walnuts
Almonds
Pumpkin Seeds
Sunflower Seeds
Sesame Seeds
Black Sesame Seeds
Olive Oil

Check if you ate:
Flaxseed Oil
Coconut Oil
Honey
Green Tea

Avoided: (Check off when you said no to)
Coffee
Sugar
Transfats
White Flour products
Alcohol
Soda
Processed Foods
Canned Foods
Diet Foods
Foods that contain transfats
Vegetable Oil and other hydrogenated oils
Soy
Products put on your body that contain chemicals
Sugar substitutes

Today's Date:

Green Foods Eaten Today:

Fruits Eaten Today:

Vegetables Eaten Today:

Nuts Eaten Today:

Seeds Eaten Today:

Healthy Oils Eaten Today:

Vegetable and/or Fruit Drinks Made Today:

Vitamin and Herb Supplements:

Glasses of high-quality, filtered or bottled water:

Check if You Ate:
Spinach
Strawberries
Broccoli
Bee Pollen
Alfalfa
Green Tea
Artichokes
Cabbage
Yams
Sweet Potatoes
Asparagus
Spirulina
Chlorella
Wheat Grass
Romaine lettuce
Seaweed
Garlic
Dandelion greens
Red peppers
Kale
Beets
Blueberries
Avocados
Apples
Pineapple
Bananas
Pomegranates
Plums
Grapes
Lemons
Brazil Nuts
Walnuts
Almonds
Pumpkin Seeds
Sunflower Seeds
Sesame Seeds
Black Sesame Seeds
Olive Oil

Check if you ate:
Flaxseed Oil
Coconut Oil
Honey
Green Tea

Avoided: (Check off when you said no to)
Coffee
Sugar
Transfats
White Flour products
Alcohol
Soda
Processed Foods
Canned Foods
Diet Foods
Foods that contain transfats
Vegetable Oil and other hydrogenated oils
Soy
Products put on your body that contain chemicals
Sugar substitutes

Today's Date:

Green Foods Eaten Today:

Fruits Eaten Today:

Vegetables Eaten Today:

Nuts Eaten Today:

Seeds Eaten Today:

Healthy Oils Eaten Today:

Vegetable and/or Fruit Drinks Made Today:

Vitamin and Herb Supplements:

Glasses of high-quality, filtered or bottled water:

Check if You Ate:

Spinach
Strawberries
Broccoli
Bee Pollen
Alfalfa
Green Tea
Artichokes
Cabbage
Yams
Sweet Potatoes
Asparagus
Spirulina
Chlorella
Wheat Grass
Romaine lettuce
Seaweed
Garlic
Dandelion greens
Red peppers
Kale
Beets
Blueberries
Avocados
Apples
Pineapple
Bananas
Pomegranates
Plums
Grapes
Lemons
Brazil Nuts
Walnuts
Almonds
Pumpkin Seeds
Sunflower Seeds
Sesame Seeds
Black Sesame Seeds
Olive Oil

Check if you ate:
Flaxseed Oil
Coconut Oil
Honey
Green Tea

Avoided: (Check off when you said no to)
Coffee
Sugar
Transfats
White Flour products
Alcohol
Soda
Processed Foods
Canned Foods
Diet Foods
Foods that contain transfats
Vegetable Oil and other hydrogenated oils
Soy
Products put on your body that contain chemicals
Sugar substitutes

Today's Date:

Green Foods Eaten Today:

Fruits Eaten Today:

Vegetables Eaten Today:

Nuts Eaten Today:

Seeds Eaten Today:

Healthy Oils Eaten Today:

Vegetable and/or Fruit Drinks Made Today:

Vitamin and Herb Supplements:

Glasses of high-quality, filtered or bottled water:

Check if You Ate:
Spinach
Strawberries
Broccoli
Bee Pollen
Alfalfa
Green Tea
Artichokes
Cabbage
Yams
Sweet Potatoes
Asparagus
Spirulina
Chlorella
Wheat Grass
Romaine lettuce
Seaweed
Garlic
Dandelion greens
Red peppers
Kale
Beets
Blueberries
Avocados
Apples
Pineapple
Bananas
Pomegranates
Plums
Grapes
Lemons
Brazil Nuts
Walnuts
Almonds
Pumpkin Seeds
Sunflower Seeds
Sesame Seeds
Black Sesame Seeds
Olive Oil

Check if you ate:
Flaxseed Oil
Coconut Oil
Honey
Green Tea

Avoided: (Check off when you said no to)
Coffee
Sugar
Transfats
White Flour products
Alcohol
Soda
Processed Foods
Canned Foods
Diet Foods
Foods that contain transfats
Vegetable Oil and other hydrogenated oils
Soy
Products put on your body that contain chemicals
Sugar substitutes

Today's Date:

Green Foods Eaten Today:

Fruits Eaten Today:

Vegetables Eaten Today:

Nuts Eaten Today:

Seeds Eaten Today:

Healthy Oils Eaten Today:

Vegetable and/or Fruit Drinks Made Today:

Vitamin and Herb Supplements:

Glasses of high-quality, filtered or bottled water:

Check if You Ate:
Spinach
Strawberries
Broccoli
Bee Pollen
Alfalfa
Green Tea
Artichokes
Cabbage
Yams
Sweet Potatoes
Asparagus
Spirulina
Chlorella
Wheat Grass
Romaine lettuce
Seaweed
Garlic
Dandelion greens
Red peppers
Kale
Beets
Blueberries
Avocados
Apples
Pineapple
Bananas
Pomegranates
Plums
Grapes
Lemons
Brazil Nuts
Walnuts
Almonds
Pumpkin Seeds
Sunflower Seeds
Sesame Seeds
Black Sesame Seeds
Olive Oil

Check if you ate:
Flaxseed Oil
Coconut Oil
Honey
Green Tea

Avoided: (Check off when you said no to)
Coffee
Sugar
Transfats
White Flour products
Alcohol
Soda
Processed Foods
Canned Foods
Diet Foods
Foods that contain transfats
Vegetable Oil and other hydrogenated oils
Soy
Products put on your body that contain chemicals
Sugar substitutes

Today's Date:

Green Foods Eaten Today:

Fruits Eaten Today:

Vegetables Eaten Today:

Nuts Eaten Today:

Seeds Eaten Today:

Healthy Oils Eaten Today:

Vegetable and/or Fruit Drinks Made Today:

Vitamin and Herb Supplements:

Glasses of high-quality, filtered or bottled water:

Check if You Ate:

Spinach
Strawberries
Broccoli
Bee Pollen
Alfalfa
Green Tea
Artichokes
Cabbage
Yams
Sweet Potatoes
Asparagus
Spirulina
Chlorella
Wheat Grass
Romaine lettuce
Seaweed
Garlic
Dandelion greens
Red peppers
Kale
Beets
Blueberries
Avocados
Apples
Pineapple
Bananas
Pomegranates
Plums
Grapes
Lemons
Brazil Nuts
Walnuts
Almonds
Pumpkin Seeds
Sunflower Seeds
Sesame Seeds
Black Sesame Seeds
Olive Oil

Check if you ate:
Flaxseed Oil
Coconut Oil
Honey
Green Tea

Avoided: (Check off when you said no to)
Coffee
Sugar
Transfats
White Flour products
Alcohol
Soda
Processed Foods
Canned Foods
Diet Foods
Foods that contain transfats
Vegetable Oil and other hydrogenated oils
Soy
Products put on your body that contain chemicals
Sugar substitutes

Today's Date:

Green Foods Eaten Today:

Fruits Eaten Today:

Vegetables Eaten Today:

Nuts Eaten Today:

Seeds Eaten Today:

Healthy Oils Eaten Today:

Vegetable and/or Fruit Drinks Made Today:

Vitamin and Herb Supplements:

Glasses of high-quality, filtered or bottled water:

Check if You Ate:
Spinach
Strawberries
Broccoli
Bee Pollen
Alfalfa
Green Tea
Artichokes
Cabbage
Yams
Sweet Potatoes
Asparagus
Spirulina
Chlorella
Wheat Grass
Romaine lettuce
Seaweed
Garlic
Dandelion greens
Red peppers
Kale
Beets
Blueberries
Avocados
Apples
Pineapple
Bananas
Pomegranates
Plums
Grapes
Lemons
Brazil Nuts
Walnuts
Almonds
Pumpkin Seeds
Sunflower Seeds
Sesame Seeds
Black Sesame Seeds
Olive Oil

Check if you ate:
Flaxseed Oil
Coconut Oil
Honey
Green Tea

Avoided: (Check off when you said no to)
Coffee
Sugar
Transfats
White Flour products
Alcohol
Soda
Processed Foods
Canned Foods
Diet Foods
Foods that contain transfats
Vegetable Oil and other hydrogenated oils
Soy
Products put on your body that contain chemicals
Sugar substitutes

Today's Date:

Green Foods Eaten Today:

Fruits Eaten Today:

Vegetables Eaten Today:

Nuts Eaten Today:

Seeds Eaten Today:

Healthy Oils Eaten Today:

Vegetable and/or Fruit Drinks Made Today:

Vitamin and Herb Supplements:

Glasses of high-quality, filtered or bottled water:

Check if You Ate:
Spinach
Strawberries
Broccoli
Bee Pollen
Alfalfa
Green Tea
Artichokes
Cabbage
Yams
Sweet Potatoes
Asparagus
Spirulina
Chlorella
Wheat Grass
Romaine lettuce
Seaweed
Garlic
Dandelion greens
Red peppers
Kale
Beets
Blueberries
Avocados
Apples
Pineapple
Bananas
Pomegranates
Plums
Grapes
Lemons
Brazil Nuts
Walnuts
Almonds
Pumpkin Seeds
Sunflower Seeds
Sesame Seeds
Black Sesame Seeds
Olive Oil

Check if you ate:
Flaxseed Oil
Coconut Oil
Honey
Green Tea

Avoided: (Check off when you said no to)
Coffee
Sugar
Transfats
White Flour products
Alcohol
Soda
Processed Foods
Canned Foods
Diet Foods
Foods that contain transfats
Vegetable Oil and other hydrogenated oils
Soy
Products put on your body that contain chemicals
Sugar substitutes

Today's Date:

Green Foods Eaten Today:

Fruits Eaten Today:

Vegetables Eaten Today:

Nuts Eaten Today:

Seeds Eaten Today:

Healthy Oils Eaten Today:

Vegetable and/or Fruit Drinks Made Today:

Vitamin and Herb Supplements:

Glasses of high-quality, filtered or bottled water:

Check if You Ate:

Spinach
Strawberries
Broccoli
Bee Pollen
Alfalfa
Green Tea
Artichokes
Cabbage
Yams
Sweet Potatoes
Asparagus
Spirulina
Chlorella
Wheat Grass
Romaine lettuce
Seaweed
Garlic
Dandelion greens
Red peppers
Kale
Beets
Blueberries
Avocados
Apples
Pineapple
Bananas
Pomegranates
Plums
Grapes
Lemons
Brazil Nuts
Walnuts
Almonds
Pumpkin Seeds
Sunflower Seeds
Sesame Seeds
Black Sesame Seeds
Olive Oil

Check if you ate:
Flaxseed Oil
Coconut Oil
Honey
Green Tea

Avoided: (Check off when you said no to)
Coffee
Sugar
Transfats
White Flour products
Alcohol
Soda
Processed Foods
Canned Foods
Diet Foods
Foods that contain transfats
Vegetable Oil and other hydrogenated oils
Soy
Products put on your body that contain chemicals
Sugar substitutes

Today's Date:

Green Foods Eaten Today:

Fruits Eaten Today:

Vegetables Eaten Today:

Nuts Eaten Today:

Seeds Eaten Today:

Healthy Oils Eaten Today:

Vegetable and/or Fruit Drinks Made Today:

Vitamin and Herb Supplements:

Glasses of high-quality, filtered or bottled water:

Check if You Ate:
Spinach
Strawberries
Broccoli
Bee Pollen
Alfalfa
Green Tea
Artichokes
Cabbage
Yams
Sweet Potatoes
Asparagus
Spirulina
Chlorella
Wheat Grass
Romaine lettuce
Seaweed
Garlic
Dandelion greens
Red peppers
Kale
Beets
Blueberries
Avocados
Apples
Pineapple
Bananas
Pomegranates
Plums
Grapes
Lemons
Brazil Nuts
Walnuts
Almonds
Pumpkin Seeds
Sunflower Seeds
Sesame Seeds
Black Sesame Seeds
Olive Oil

Check if you ate:
Flaxseed Oil
Coconut Oil
Honey
Green Tea

Avoided: (Check off when you said no to)
Coffee
Sugar
Transfats
White Flour products
Alcohol
Soda
Processed Foods
Canned Foods
Diet Foods
Foods that contain transfats
Vegetable Oil and other hydrogenated oils
Soy
Products put on your body that contain chemicals
Sugar substitutes

Today's Date:

Green Foods Eaten Today:

Fruits Eaten Today:

Vegetables Eaten Today:

Nuts Eaten Today:

Seeds Eaten Today:

Healthy Oils Eaten Today:

Vegetable and/or Fruit Drinks Made Today:

Vitamin and Herb Supplements:

Glasses of high-quality, filtered or bottled water:

Check if You Ate:
Spinach
Strawberries
Broccoli
Bee Pollen
Alfalfa
Green Tea
Artichokes
Cabbage
Yams
Sweet Potatoes
Asparagus
Spirulina
Chlorella
Wheat Grass
Romaine lettuce
Seaweed
Garlic
Dandelion greens
Red peppers
Kale
Beets
Blueberries
Avocados
Apples
Pineapple
Bananas
Pomegranates
Plums
Grapes
Lemons
Brazil Nuts
Walnuts
Almonds
Pumpkin Seeds
Sunflower Seeds
Sesame Seeds
Black Sesame Seeds
Olive Oil

Check if you ate:
Flaxseed Oil
Coconut Oil
Honey
Green Tea

Avoided: (Check off when you said no to)
Coffee
Sugar
Transfats
White Flour products
Alcohol
Soda
Processed Foods
Canned Foods
Diet Foods
Foods that contain transfats
Vegetable Oil and other hydrogenated oils
Soy
Products put on your body that contain chemicals
Sugar substitutes

Today's Date:

Green Foods Eaten Today:

Fruits Eaten Today:

Vegetables Eaten Today:

Nuts Eaten Today:

Seeds Eaten Today:

Healthy Oils Eaten Today:

Vegetable and/or Fruit Drinks Made Today:

Vitamin and Herb Supplements:

Glasses of high-quality, filtered or bottled water:

Check if You Ate:
Spinach
Strawberries
Broccoli
Bee Pollen
Alfalfa
Green Tea
Artichokes
Cabbage
Yams
Sweet Potatoes
Asparagus
Spirulina
Chlorella
Wheat Grass
Romaine lettuce
Seaweed
Garlic
Dandelion greens
Red peppers
Kale
Beets
Blueberries
Avocados
Apples
Pineapple
Bananas
Pomegranates
Plums
Grapes
Lemons
Brazil Nuts
Walnuts
Almonds
Pumpkin Seeds
Sunflower Seeds
Sesame Seeds
Black Sesame Seeds
Olive Oil

Check if you ate:
Flaxseed Oil
Coconut Oil
Honey
Green Tea

Avoided: (Check off when you said no to)
Coffee
Sugar
Transfats
White Flour products
Alcohol
Soda
Processed Foods
Canned Foods
Diet Foods
Foods that contain transfats
Vegetable Oil and other hydrogenated oils
Soy
Products put on your body that contain chemicals
Sugar substitutes

Today's Date:

Green Foods Eaten Today:

Fruits Eaten Today:

Vegetables Eaten Today:

Nuts Eaten Today:

Seeds Eaten Today:

Healthy Oils Eaten Today:

Vegetable and/or Fruit Drinks Made Today:

Vitamin and Herb Supplements:

Glasses of high-quality, filtered or bottled water:

Check if You Ate:
Spinach
Strawberries
Broccoli
Bee Pollen
Alfalfa
Green Tea
Artichokes
Cabbage
Yams
Sweet Potatoes
Asparagus
Spirulina
Chlorella
Wheat Grass
Romaine lettuce
Seaweed
Garlic
Dandelion greens
Red peppers
Kale
Beets
Blueberries
Avocados
Apples
Pineapple
Bananas
Pomegranates
Plums
Grapes
Lemons
Brazil Nuts
Walnuts
Almonds
Pumpkin Seeds
Sunflower Seeds
Sesame Seeds
Black Sesame Seeds
Olive Oil

Check if you ate:
Flaxseed Oil
Coconut Oil
Honey
Green Tea

Avoided: (Check off when you said no to)
Coffee
Sugar
Transfats
White Flour products
Alcohol
Soda
Processed Foods
Canned Foods
Diet Foods
Foods that contain transfats
Vegetable Oil and other hydrogenated oils
Soy
Products put on your body that contain chemicals
Sugar substitutes

Today's Date:

Green Foods Eaten Today:

Fruits Eaten Today:

Vegetables Eaten Today:

Nuts Eaten Today:

Seeds Eaten Today:

Healthy Oils Eaten Today:

Vegetable and/or Fruit Drinks Made Today:

Vitamin and Herb Supplements:

Glasses of high-quality, filtered or bottled water:

Check if You Ate:
Spinach
Strawberries
Broccoli
Bee Pollen
Alfalfa
Green Tea
Artichokes
Cabbage
Yams
Sweet Potatoes
Asparagus
Spirulina
Chlorella
Wheat Grass
Romaine lettuce
Seaweed
Garlic
Dandelion greens
Red peppers
Kale
Beets
Blueberries
Avocados
Apples
Pineapple
Bananas
Pomegranates
Plums
Grapes
Lemons
Brazil Nuts
Walnuts
Almonds
Pumpkin Seeds
Sunflower Seeds
Sesame Seeds
Black Sesame Seeds
Olive Oil

Check if you ate:
Flaxseed Oil
Coconut Oil
Honey
Green Tea

Avoided: (Check off when you said no to)
Coffee
Sugar
Transfats
White Flour products
Alcohol
Soda
Processed Foods
Canned Foods
Diet Foods
Foods that contain transfats
Vegetable Oil and other hydrogenated oils
Soy
Products put on your body that contain chemicals
Sugar substitutes

Today's Date:

Green Foods Eaten Today:

Fruits Eaten Today:

Vegetables Eaten Today:

Nuts Eaten Today:

Seeds Eaten Today:

Healthy Oils Eaten Today:

Vegetable and/or Fruit Drinks Made Today:

Vitamin and Herb Supplements:

Glasses of high-quality, filtered or bottled water:

Check if You Ate:

Spinach
Strawberries
Broccoli
Bee Pollen
Alfalfa
Green Tea
Artichokes
Cabbage
Yams
Sweet Potatoes
Asparagus
Spirulina
Chlorella
Wheat Grass
Romaine lettuce
Seaweed
Garlic
Dandelion greens
Red peppers
Kale
Beets
Blueberries
Avocados
Apples
Pineapple
Bananas
Pomegranates
Plums
Grapes
Lemons
Brazil Nuts
Walnuts
Almonds
Pumpkin Seeds
Sunflower Seeds
Sesame Seeds
Black Sesame Seeds
Olive Oil

Check if you ate:
Flaxseed Oil
Coconut Oil
Honey
Green Tea

Avoided: (Check off when you said no to)
Coffee
Sugar
Transfats
White Flour products
Alcohol
Soda
Processed Foods
Canned Foods
Diet Foods
Foods that contain transfats
Vegetable Oil and other hydrogenated oils
Soy
Products put on your body that contain chemicals
Sugar substitutes

Today's Date:

Green Foods Eaten Today:

Fruits Eaten Today:

Vegetables Eaten Today:

Nuts Eaten Today:

Seeds Eaten Today:

Healthy Oils Eaten Today:

Vegetable and/or Fruit Drinks Made Today:

Vitamin and Herb Supplements:

Glasses of high-quality, filtered or bottled water:

Check if You Ate:
Spinach
Strawberries
Broccoli
Bee Pollen
Alfalfa
Green Tea
Artichokes
Cabbage
Yams
Sweet Potatoes
Asparagus
Spirulina
Chlorella
Wheat Grass
Romaine lettuce
Seaweed
Garlic
Dandelion greens
Red peppers
Kale
Beets
Blueberries
Avocados
Apples
Pineapple
Bananas
Pomegranates
Plums
Grapes
Lemons
Brazil Nuts
Walnuts
Almonds
Pumpkin Seeds
Sunflower Seeds
Sesame Seeds
Black Sesame Seeds
Olive Oil

Check if you ate:
Flaxseed Oil
Coconut Oil
Honey
Green Tea

Avoided: (Check off when you said no to)
Coffee
Sugar
Transfats
White Flour products
Alcohol
Soda
Processed Foods
Canned Foods
Diet Foods
Foods that contain transfats
Vegetable Oil and other hydrogenated oils
Soy
Products put on your body that contain chemicals
Sugar substitutes

Today's Date:

Green Foods Eaten Today:

Fruits Eaten Today:

Vegetables Eaten Today:

Nuts Eaten Today:

Seeds Eaten Today:

Healthy Oils Eaten Today:

Vegetable and/or Fruit Drinks Made Today:

Vitamin and Herb Supplements:

Glasses of high-quality, filtered or bottled water:

Check if You Ate:
Spinach
Strawberries
Broccoli
Bee Pollen
Alfalfa
Green Tea
Artichokes
Cabbage
Yams
Sweet Potatoes
Asparagus
Spirulina
Chlorella
Wheat Grass
Romaine lettuce
Seaweed
Garlic
Dandelion greens
Red peppers
Kale
Beets
Blueberries
Avocados
Apples
Pineapple
Bananas
Pomegranates
Plums
Grapes
Lemons
Brazil Nuts
Walnuts
Almonds
Pumpkin Seeds
Sunflower Seeds
Sesame Seeds
Black Sesame Seeds
Olive Oil

Check if you ate:
Flaxseed Oil
Coconut Oil
Honey
Green Tea

Avoided: (Check off when you said no to)
Coffee
Sugar
Transfats
White Flour products
Alcohol
Soda
Processed Foods
Canned Foods
Diet Foods
Foods that contain transfats
Vegetable Oil and other hydrogenated oils
Soy
Products put on your body that contain chemicals
Sugar substitutes

Today's Date:

Green Foods Eaten Today:

Fruits Eaten Today:

Vegetables Eaten Today:

Nuts Eaten Today:

Seeds Eaten Today:

Healthy Oils Eaten Today:

Vegetable and/or Fruit Drinks Made Today:

Vitamin and Herb Supplements:

Glasses of high-quality, filtered or bottled water:

Check if You Ate:
Spinach
Strawberries
Broccoli
Bee Pollen
Alfalfa
Green Tea
Artichokes
Cabbage
Yams
Sweet Potatoes
Asparagus
Spirulina
Chlorella
Wheat Grass
Romaine lettuce
Seaweed
Garlic
Dandelion greens
Red peppers
Kale
Beets
Blueberries
Avocados
Apples
Pineapple
Bananas
Pomegranates
Plums
Grapes
Lemons
Brazil Nuts
Walnuts
Almonds
Pumpkin Seeds
Sunflower Seeds
Sesame Seeds
Black Sesame Seeds
Olive Oil

Check if you ate:
Flaxseed Oil
Coconut Oil
Honey
Green Tea

Avoided: (Check off when you said no to)
Coffee
Sugar
Transfats
White Flour products
Alcohol
Soda
Processed Foods
Canned Foods
Diet Foods
Foods that contain transfats
Vegetable Oil and other hydrogenated oils
Soy
Products put on your body that contain chemicals
Sugar substitutes

Today's Date:

Green Foods Eaten Today:

Fruits Eaten Today:

Vegetables Eaten Today:

Nuts Eaten Today:

Seeds Eaten Today:

Healthy Oils Eaten Today:

Vegetable and/or Fruit Drinks Made Today:

Vitamin and Herb Supplements:

Glasses of high-quality, filtered or bottled water:

Check if You Ate:
Spinach
Strawberries
Broccoli
Bee Pollen
Alfalfa
Green Tea
Artichokes
Cabbage
Yams
Sweet Potatoes
Asparagus
Spirulina
Chlorella
Wheat Grass
Romaine lettuce
Seaweed
Garlic
Dandelion greens
Red peppers
Kale
Beets
Blueberries
Avocados
Apples
Pineapple
Bananas
Pomegranates
Plums
Grapes
Lemons
Brazil Nuts
Walnuts
Almonds
Pumpkin Seeds
Sunflower Seeds
Sesame Seeds
Black Sesame Seeds
Olive Oil

Check if you ate:
Flaxseed Oil
Coconut Oil
Honey
Green Tea

Avoided: (Check off when you said no to)
Coffee
Sugar
Transfats
White Flour products
Alcohol
Soda
Processed Foods
Canned Foods
Diet Foods
Foods that contain transfats
Vegetable Oil and other hydrogenated oils
Soy
Products put on your body that contain chemicals
Sugar substitutes

Today's Date:

Green Foods Eaten Today:

Fruits Eaten Today:

Vegetables Eaten Today:

Nuts Eaten Today:

Seeds Eaten Today:

Healthy Oils Eaten Today:

Vegetable and/or Fruit Drinks Made Today:

Vitamin and Herb Supplements:

Glasses of high-quality, filtered or bottled water:

Check if You Ate:
Spinach
Strawberries
Broccoli
Bee Pollen
Alfalfa
Green Tea
Artichokes
Cabbage
Yams
Sweet Potatoes
Asparagus
Spirulina
Chlorella
Wheat Grass
Romaine lettuce
Seaweed
Garlic
Dandelion greens
Red peppers
Kale
Beets
Blueberries
Avocados
Apples
Pineapple
Bananas
Pomegranates
Plums
Grapes
Lemons
Brazil Nuts
Walnuts
Almonds
Pumpkin Seeds
Sunflower Seeds
Sesame Seeds
Black Sesame Seeds
Olive Oil

Check if you ate:
Flaxseed Oil
Coconut Oil
Honey
Green Tea

Avoided: (Check off when you said no to)
Coffee
Sugar
Transfats
White Flour products
Alcohol
Soda
Processed Foods
Canned Foods
Diet Foods
Foods that contain transfats
Vegetable Oil and other hydrogenated oils
Soy
Products put on your body that contain chemicals
Sugar substitutes

Today's Date:

Green Foods Eaten Today:

Fruits Eaten Today:

Vegetables Eaten Today:

Nuts Eaten Today:

Seeds Eaten Today:

Healthy Oils Eaten Today:

Vegetable and/or Fruit Drinks Made Today:

Vitamin and Herb Supplements:

Glasses of high-quality, filtered or bottled water:

Check if You Ate:

Spinach
Strawberries
Broccoli
Bee Pollen
Alfalfa
Green Tea
Artichokes
Cabbage
Yams
Sweet Potatoes
Asparagus
Spirulina
Chlorella
Wheat Grass
Romaine lettuce
Seaweed
Garlic
Dandelion greens
Red peppers
Kale
Beets
Blueberries
Avocados
Apples
Pineapple
Bananas
Pomegranates
Plums
Grapes
Lemons
Brazil Nuts
Walnuts
Almonds
Pumpkin Seeds
Sunflower Seeds
Sesame Seeds
Black Sesame Seeds
Olive Oil

Check if you ate:
Flaxseed Oil
Coconut Oil
Honey
Green Tea

Avoided: (Check off when you said no to)
Coffee
Sugar
Transfats
White Flour products
Alcohol
Soda
Processed Foods
Canned Foods
Diet Foods
Foods that contain transfats
Vegetable Oil and other hydrogenated oils
Soy
Products put on your body that contain chemicals
Sugar substitutes

Today's Date:

Green Foods Eaten Today:

Fruits Eaten Today:

Vegetables Eaten Today:

Nuts Eaten Today:

Seeds Eaten Today:

Healthy Oils Eaten Today:

Vegetable and/or Fruit Drinks Made Today:

Vitamin and Herb Supplements:

Glasses of high-quality, filtered or bottled water:

Check if You Ate:
Spinach
Strawberries
Broccoli
Bee Pollen
Alfalfa
Green Tea
Artichokes
Cabbage
Yams
Sweet Potatoes
Asparagus
Spirulina
Chlorella
Wheat Grass
Romaine lettuce
Seaweed
Garlic
Dandelion greens
Red peppers
Kale
Beets
Blueberries
Avocados
Apples
Pineapple
Bananas
Pomegranates
Plums
Grapes
Lemons
Brazil Nuts
Walnuts
Almonds
Pumpkin Seeds
Sunflower Seeds
Sesame Seeds
Black Sesame Seeds
Olive Oil

Check if you ate:
Flaxseed Oil
Coconut Oil
Honey
Green Tea

Avoided: (Check off when you said no to)
Coffee
Sugar
Transfats
White Flour products
Alcohol
Soda
Processed Foods
Canned Foods
Diet Foods
Foods that contain transfats
Vegetable Oil and other hydrogenated oils
Soy
Products put on your body that contain chemicals
Sugar substitutes

Today's Date:

Green Foods Eaten Today:

Fruits Eaten Today:

Vegetables Eaten Today:

Nuts Eaten Today:

Seeds Eaten Today:

Healthy Oils Eaten Today:

Vegetable and/or Fruit Drinks Made Today:

Vitamin and Herb Supplements:

Glasses of high-quality, filtered or bottled water:

Check if You Ate:

Spinach
Strawberries
Broccoli
Bee Pollen
Alfalfa
Green Tea
Artichokes
Cabbage
Yams
Sweet Potatoes
Asparagus
Spirulina
Chlorella
Wheat Grass
Romaine lettuce
Seaweed
Garlic
Dandelion greens
Red peppers
Kale
Beets
Blueberries
Avocados
Apples
Pineapple
Bananas
Pomegranates
Plums
Grapes
Lemons
Brazil Nuts
Walnuts
Almonds
Pumpkin Seeds
Sunflower Seeds
Sesame Seeds
Black Sesame Seeds
Olive Oil

Check if you ate:
Flaxseed Oil
Coconut Oil
Honey
Green Tea

Avoided: (Check off when you said no to)
Coffee
Sugar
Transfats
White Flour products
Alcohol
Soda
Processed Foods
Canned Foods
Diet Foods
Foods that contain transfats
Vegetable Oil and other hydrogenated oils
Soy
Products put on your body that contain chemicals
Sugar substitutes

Today's Date:

Green Foods Eaten Today:

Fruits Eaten Today:

Vegetables Eaten Today:

Nuts Eaten Today:

Seeds Eaten Today:

Healthy Oils Eaten Today:

Vegetable and/or Fruit Drinks Made Today:

Vitamin and Herb Supplements:

Glasses of high-quality, filtered or bottled water:

Check if You Ate:
Spinach
Strawberries
Broccoli
Bee Pollen
Alfalfa
Green Tea
Artichokes
Cabbage
Yams
Sweet Potatoes
Asparagus
Spirulina
Chlorella
Wheat Grass
Romaine lettuce
Seaweed
Garlic
Dandelion greens
Red peppers
Kale
Beets
Blueberries
Avocados
Apples
Pineapple
Bananas
Pomegranates
Plums
Grapes
Lemons
Brazil Nuts
Walnuts
Almonds
Pumpkin Seeds
Sunflower Seeds
Sesame Seeds
Black Sesame Seeds
Olive Oil

Check if you ate:
Flaxseed Oil
Coconut Oil
Honey
Green Tea

Avoided: (Check off when you said no to)
Coffee
Sugar
Transfats
White Flour products
Alcohol
Soda
Processed Foods
Canned Foods
Diet Foods
Foods that contain transfats
Vegetable Oil and other hydrogenated oils
Soy
Products put on your body that contain chemicals
Sugar substitutes

Today's Date:

Green Foods Eaten Today:

Fruits Eaten Today:

Vegetables Eaten Today:

Nuts Eaten Today:

Seeds Eaten Today:

Healthy Oils Eaten Today:

Vegetable and/or Fruit Drinks Made Today:

Vitamin and Herb Supplements:

Glasses of high-quality, filtered or bottled water:

Check if You Ate:
Spinach
Strawberries
Broccoli
Bee Pollen
Alfalfa
Green Tea
Artichokes
Cabbage
Yams
Sweet Potatoes
Asparagus
Spirulina
Chlorella
Wheat Grass
Romaine lettuce
Seaweed
Garlic
Dandelion greens
Red peppers
Kale
Beets
Blueberries
Avocados
Apples
Pineapple
Bananas
Pomegranates
Plums
Grapes
Lemons
Brazil Nuts
Walnuts
Almonds
Pumpkin Seeds
Sunflower Seeds
Sesame Seeds
Black Sesame Seeds
Olive Oil

Check if you ate:
Flaxseed Oil
Coconut Oil
Honey
Green Tea

Avoided: (Check off when you said no to)
Coffee
Sugar
Transfats
White Flour products
Alcohol
Soda
Processed Foods
Canned Foods
Diet Foods
Foods that contain transfats
Vegetable Oil and other hydrogenated oils
Soy
Products put on your body that contain chemicals
Sugar substitutes

Today's Date:

Green Foods Eaten Today:

Fruits Eaten Today:

Vegetables Eaten Today:

Nuts Eaten Today:

Seeds Eaten Today:

Healthy Oils Eaten Today:

Vegetable and/or Fruit Drinks Made Today:

Vitamin and Herb Supplements:

Glasses of high-quality, filtered or bottled water:

Check if You Ate:
Spinach
Strawberries
Broccoli
Bee Pollen
Alfalfa
Green Tea
Artichokes
Cabbage
Yams
Sweet Potatoes
Asparagus
Spirulina
Chlorella
Wheat Grass
Romaine lettuce
Seaweed
Garlic
Dandelion greens
Red peppers
Kale
Beets
Blueberries
Avocados
Apples
Pineapple
Bananas
Pomegranates
Plums
Grapes
Lemons
Brazil Nuts
Walnuts
Almonds
Pumpkin Seeds
Sunflower Seeds
Sesame Seeds
Black Sesame Seeds
Olive Oil

Check if you ate:
Flaxseed Oil
Coconut Oil
Honey
Green Tea

Avoided: (Check off when you said no to)
Coffee
Sugar
Transfats
White Flour products
Alcohol
Soda
Processed Foods
Canned Foods
Diet Foods
Foods that contain transfats
Vegetable Oil and other hydrogenated oils
Soy
Products put on your body that contain chemicals
Sugar substitutes

Today's Date:

Green Foods Eaten Today:

Fruits Eaten Today:

Vegetables Eaten Today:

Nuts Eaten Today:

Seeds Eaten Today:

Healthy Oils Eaten Today:

Vegetable and/or Fruit Drinks Made Today:

Vitamin and Herb Supplements:

Glasses of high-quality, filtered or bottled water:

Check if You Ate:
Spinach
Strawberries
Broccoli
Bee Pollen
Alfalfa
Green Tea
Artichokes
Cabbage
Yams
Sweet Potatoes
Asparagus
Spirulina
Chlorella
Wheat Grass
Romaine lettuce
Seaweed
Garlic
Dandelion greens
Red peppers
Kale
Beets
Blueberries
Avocados
Apples
Pineapple
Bananas
Pomegranates
Plums
Grapes
Lemons
Brazil Nuts
Walnuts
Almonds
Pumpkin Seeds
Sunflower Seeds
Sesame Seeds
Black Sesame Seeds
Olive Oil

Check if you ate:
Flaxseed Oil
Coconut Oil
Honey
Green Tea

Avoided: (Check off when you said no to)
Coffee
Sugar
Transfats
White Flour products
Alcohol
Soda
Processed Foods
Canned Foods
Diet Foods
Foods that contain transfats
Vegetable Oil and other hydrogenated oils
Soy
Products put on your body that contain chemicals
Sugar substitutes

Today's Date:

Green Foods Eaten Today:

Fruits Eaten Today:

Vegetables Eaten Today:

Nuts Eaten Today:

Seeds Eaten Today:

Healthy Oils Eaten Today:

Vegetable and/or Fruit Drinks Made Today:

Vitamin and Herb Supplements:

Glasses of high-quality, filtered or bottled water:

Check if You Ate:
Spinach
Strawberries
Broccoli
Bee Pollen
Alfalfa
Green Tea
Artichokes
Cabbage
Yams
Sweet Potatoes
Asparagus
Spirulina
Chlorella
Wheat Grass
Romaine lettuce
Seaweed
Garlic
Dandelion greens
Red peppers
Kale
Beets
Blueberries
Avocados
Apples
Pineapple
Bananas
Pomegranates
Plums
Grapes
Lemons
Brazil Nuts
Walnuts
Almonds
Pumpkin Seeds
Sunflower Seeds
Sesame Seeds
Black Sesame Seeds
Olive Oil

Check if you ate:
Flaxseed Oil
Coconut Oil
Honey
Green Tea

Avoided: (Check off when you said no to)
Coffee
Sugar
Transfats
White Flour products
Alcohol
Soda
Processed Foods
Canned Foods
Diet Foods
Foods that contain transfats
Vegetable Oil and other hydrogenated oils
Soy
Products put on your body that contain chemicals
Sugar substitutes

Today's Date:

Green Foods Eaten Today:

Fruits Eaten Today:

Vegetables Eaten Today:

Nuts Eaten Today:

Seeds Eaten Today:

Healthy Oils Eaten Today:

Vegetable and/or Fruit Drinks Made Today:

Vitamin and Herb Supplements:

Glasses of high-quality, filtered or bottled water:

Check if You Ate:
Spinach
Strawberries
Broccoli
Bee Pollen
Alfalfa
Green Tea
Artichokes
Cabbage
Yams
Sweet Potatoes
Asparagus
Spirulina
Chlorella
Wheat Grass
Romaine lettuce
Seaweed
Garlic
Dandelion greens
Red peppers
Kale
Beets
Blueberries
Avocados
Apples
Pineapple
Bananas
Pomegranates
Plums
Grapes
Lemons
Brazil Nuts
Walnuts
Almonds
Pumpkin Seeds
Sunflower Seeds
Sesame Seeds
Black Sesame Seeds
Olive Oil

Check if you ate:
Flaxseed Oil
Coconut Oil
Honey
Green Tea

Avoided: (Check off when you said no to)
Coffee
Sugar
Transfats
White Flour products
Alcohol
Soda
Processed Foods
Canned Foods
Diet Foods
Foods that contain transfats
Vegetable Oil and other hydrogenated oils
Soy
Products put on your body that contain chemicals
Sugar substitutes

Today's Date:

Green Foods Eaten Today:

Fruits Eaten Today:

Vegetables Eaten Today:

Nuts Eaten Today:

Seeds Eaten Today:

Healthy Oils Eaten Today:

Vegetable and/or Fruit Drinks Made Today:

Vitamin and Herb Supplements:

Glasses of high-quality, filtered or bottled water:

Check if You Ate:
Spinach
Strawberries
Broccoli
Bee Pollen
Alfalfa
Green Tea
Artichokes
Cabbage
Yams
Sweet Potatoes
Asparagus
Spirulina
Chlorella
Wheat Grass
Romaine lettuce
Seaweed
Garlic
Dandelion greens
Red peppers
Kale
Beets
Blueberries
Avocados
Apples
Pineapple
Bananas
Pomegranates
Plums
Grapes
Lemons
Brazil Nuts
Walnuts
Almonds
Pumpkin Seeds
Sunflower Seeds
Sesame Seeds
Black Sesame Seeds
Olive Oil

Check if you ate:
Flaxseed Oil
Coconut Oil
Honey
Green Tea

Avoided: (Check off when you said no to)
Coffee
Sugar
Transfats
White Flour products
Alcohol
Soda
Processed Foods
Canned Foods
Diet Foods
Foods that contain transfats
Vegetable Oil and other hydrogenated oils
Soy
Products put on your body that contain chemicals
Sugar substitutes

Today's Date:

Green Foods Eaten Today:

Fruits Eaten Today:

Vegetables Eaten Today:

Nuts Eaten Today:

Seeds Eaten Today:

Healthy Oils Eaten Today:

Vegetable and/or Fruit Drinks Made Today:

Vitamin and Herb Supplements:

Glasses of high-quality, filtered or bottled water:

Check if You Ate:
Spinach
Strawberries
Broccoli
Bee Pollen
Alfalfa
Green Tea
Artichokes
Cabbage
Yams
Sweet Potatoes
Asparagus
Spirulina
Chlorella
Wheat Grass
Romaine lettuce
Seaweed
Garlic
Dandelion greens
Red peppers
Kale
Beets
Blueberries
Avocados
Apples
Pineapple
Bananas
Pomegranates
Plums
Grapes
Lemons
Brazil Nuts
Walnuts
Almonds
Pumpkin Seeds
Sunflower Seeds
Sesame Seeds
Black Sesame Seeds
Olive Oil

Check if you ate:
Flaxseed Oil
Coconut Oil
Honey
Green Tea

Avoided: (Check off when you said no to)
Coffee
Sugar
Transfats
White Flour products
Alcohol
Soda
Processed Foods
Canned Foods
Diet Foods
Foods that contain transfats
Vegetable Oil and other hydrogenated oils
Soy
Products put on your body that contain chemicals
Sugar substitutes

Today's Date:

Green Foods Eaten Today:

Fruits Eaten Today:

Vegetables Eaten Today:

Nuts Eaten Today:

Seeds Eaten Today:

Healthy Oils Eaten Today:

Vegetable and/or Fruit Drinks Made Today:

Vitamin and Herb Supplements:

Glasses of high-quality, filtered or bottled water:

Check if You Ate:
Spinach
Strawberries
Broccoli
Bee Pollen
Alfalfa
Green Tea
Artichokes
Cabbage
Yams
Sweet Potatoes
Asparagus
Spirulina
Chlorella
Wheat Grass
Romaine lettuce
Seaweed
Garlic
Dandelion greens
Red peppers
Kale
Beets
Blueberries
Avocados
Apples
Pineapple
Bananas
Pomegranates
Plums
Grapes
Lemons
Brazil Nuts
Walnuts
Almonds
Pumpkin Seeds
Sunflower Seeds
Sesame Seeds
Black Sesame Seeds
Olive Oil

Check if you ate:
Flaxseed Oil
Coconut Oil
Honey
Green Tea

Avoided: (Check off when you said no to)
Coffee
Sugar
Transfats
White Flour products
Alcohol
Soda
Processed Foods
Canned Foods
Diet Foods
Foods that contain transfats
Vegetable Oil and other hydrogenated oils
Soy
Products put on your body that contain chemicals
Sugar substitutes